Healing Hands, Guided Hearts: Daily Devotionals for Christian Doctors

Delightful Devotionals

CONTENTS

Introduction

In the realm of medicine, where science and compassion converge, a doctor's journey is both an art and a calling. The heartbeat of healing resonates with God's plan for humanity—a rhythm that pulsates through every diagnosis, every treatment, and every encounter with those seeking relief in the face of illness.

This collection of devotionals is designed specifically for the healers of this world, our doctors, each day's reflection is an invitation to pause, reflect, and draw strength from the wellspring of faith.

As you embark on this beautiful exploration, consider it a respite for the healer's heart. Each verse, reflection, and encouragement is crafted to nurture the spiritual dimensions of your journey. From the divine gift of healing hands to the delicate balance between science and faith, this collection offers a moment of divine reflection for doctors navigating the intricate landscapes of medicine.

The demands of the medical profession can be intense, and the challenges faced can be daunting. Yet, within these pages, you'll find a sanctuary—a place to renew your spirit, draw inspiration from the Word, and discover the timeless wisdom that accompanies the path of a doctor.

May this collection be a guiding light, providing comfort and strength as you navigate the complexities of medical practice. As you delve into these devotionals, may your journey be enriched, your heart be fortified, and your purpose as a healer be illuminated by the divine grace that transcends both the art and science of medicine.

Day 1: Healing Hands

Verse of the Day:

Verse: Jeremiah 30:17 (NIV) - "But I will restore you to health and heal your wounds, declares the Lord because you are called an outcast, Zion for whom no one cares."

Reflection:

As a healer, you carry a divine gift – the ability to mend wounds and bring restoration. The promise in Jeremiah 30:17 echoes God's commitment to bringing healing to those who are hurting.

In your hands, you hold the instruments not only of medical skill but also of God's compassion and restoration.

Reflect on the profound responsibility that comes with being a conduit of healing. Your hands are guided not only by medical knowledge but by the divine intention to bring wholeness to those in need. Consider the impact of your healing touch, not just on physical ailments but on the deeper wounds of the soul.

In the process of mending others, take a moment to recognize that God is the ultimate healer. Your hands are an extension of His grace and mercy, instruments through which He fulfills His promise of restoration. May every patient you touch experience a glimpse of God's love through the healing journey.

Encouragement:

In your hands, God has placed the power to bring about transformation. Trust that, just as He declares in Jeremiah, He will restore health and heal wounds through your dedication and skill. Your work is not only a profession but a divine calling, and God is with you in every step of the healing process.

Journal:

1. How do you perceive the connection between your healing work and God's promise of restoration in Jeremiah 30:17?

2. Reflect on a specific instance where you witnessed not just physical healing but a deeper emotional, or spiritual healing in a patient. What impact did it have on you?

3. In what ways can you intentionally incorporate a sense of God's compassion into your daily practice of healing, recognizing that you are an instrument of His grace?

Day 2: The Physician's Compassion

Verse of the Day:

Colossians 3:12 (NIV) - "Therefore, as God's chosen people, holy and dearly loved, clothe yourselves with compassion, kindness, humility, gentleness, and patience."

Reflection:

As we delve into the second day of our journey, let's center our thoughts on the profound quality of compassion.

The verse from Colossians 3:12 not only reminds us of our calling as God's chosen people but also instructs us to clothe ourselves with compassion, mirroring God's boundless love.

For a physician, compassion is more than a virtue—it's a transformative force that fosters healing and embodies the very nature of God.

Reflect on the instances in your medical practice where compassion played a pivotal role. Consider the times when a kind word, a listening ear, or a comforting presence made a difference in a patient's journey.In these moments, you echo the divine compassion described in Colossians, becoming a living testament to the love of the Great Physician.

Encouragement:

Dear physician, your practice of compassion is a reflection of the divine love that envelops each patient you encounter. Just as God's compassion knows no bounds, may your heart overflow with empathy and kindness. Embrace the understanding that, in your compassionate care, you are not only treating ailments but also contributing to the holistic well-being of those entrusted to you.

Journal:

1. Recollect a specific patient interaction where compassion played a significant role. How did that experience impact both you and the patient?

2. In what ways do you currently integrate compassion into your medical practice? Are there areas where you can further cultivate this virtue?

3. Consider the attributes listed in Colossians 3:12, including compassion, kindness, humility, gentleness, and patience. How can incorporating these qualities enhance your effectiveness as a physician and deepen the impact of your care?

15

Day 3: Divine Diagnosis

Verse of the Day:

James 1:5 (NIV) - "If any of you lacks wisdom, you should ask God, who gives generously to all without finding fault, and it will be given to you."

Reflection:

In the intricate realm of medicine, the ability to make accurate diagnoses is both a skill and a divine gift. James 1:5 reminds us of the divine source of wisdom. As a physician, seeking divine guidance in diagnosis is an acknowledgment that true wisdom comes from God.

Reflect on the moments when the complexity of a medical case required more than your knowledge and experience. Consider the times you sought divine wisdom, either consciously or intuitively, and how it influenced your diagnosis and treatment plan.

Understanding that God grants wisdom generously without finding fault allows you to approach your diagnostic role with humility. It's an invitation to partner with the Divine Physician, trusting that in seeking His wisdom, you contribute to the healing journey of those under your care.

Encouragement:

In your pursuit of diagnostic accuracy, embrace the promise of James 1:5. God's wisdom is available to guide your discernment, refine your diagnostic skills, and lead you to effective treatment strategies. Your commitment to seeking divine insight reflects not only professional diligence but also a reliance on the ultimate source of wisdom.

Journal:

1. Can you recall a specific instance in your medical practice where seeking divine wisdom played a crucial role in making a diagnosis or treatment decision?

2. How does the promise in James 1:5 impact your approach to the challenges and uncertainties in diagnostic medicine?

3. In what ways can you integrate intentional moments of seeking God's wisdom into your daily routine as a healthcare professional?

18

Day 4: The Burden Bearer

Verse of the Day:

Psalm 55:22 (NIV) - "Cast your cares on the Lord and he will sustain you; he will never let the righteous be shaken."

Reflection:

In the noble pursuit of healing, doctors often carry the weight of their patients' physical and emotional burdens. Psalm 55:22 extends a profound invitation to cast these cares upon the Lord, the ultimate Burden Bearer. As a doctor, reflecting on the emotional and physical toll of your profession and surrendering these burdens to God is an essential practice.

Consider the burdens you've encountered in your medical career—the difficult diagnoses, the emotional toll of patient care, and the weight of responsibility. Reflect on how casting these cares upon the Lord brings a sense of sustenance and relief. The divine promise is that He will sustain you, providing strength and resilience.

Encouragement:

Doctor, acknowledge the weight you carry and find solace in the comforting arms of the Lord. In casting your burdens upon Him, you embrace the promise of sustaining grace. Recognize that seeking refuge in God's strength is not a sign of weakness but a testament to your reliance on the ultimate Burden Bearer.

Journal:

1. What burdens or challenges in your medical practice have felt particularly heavy recently? How might casting these cares upon the Lord bring you a sense of sustenance?

2. Reflect on a specific instance where surrendering a burden to God brought you peace and strength. How did this experience impact your ability to navigate challenges in your profession?

3. Consider developing a ritual of surrendering your burdens to God regularly. How can you incorporate moments of prayer or reflection into your routine to cast your cares upon the ultimate Burden Bearer?

Day 5: Restoring Hope

Verse of the Day:

Romans 15:13 (NIV) - "May the God of hope fill you with all joy and peace as you trust in him, so that you may overflow with hope by the power of the Holy Spirit."

Reflection:

Restoring hope is a sacred calling within the realm of medicine. Romans 15:13 beautifully expresses the divine source of hope and the transformative power it holds. As a healthcare provider, you are not just a practitioner of medicine; you are a bearer of hope, a conduit for the God of hope to work through.

Reflect on instances in your medical practice where you witnessed the restoration of hope. Consider the times when the healing journey extended beyond the physical, bringing joy and peace to those under your care.

The verse reminds us that our ability to restore hope is intrinsically connected to our trust in the God of hope. Explore how cultivating trust in God impacts your capacity to instill hope in your patients, colleagues, and even within yourself during challenging moments.

Encouragement:

In the midst of medical challenges, may you find encouragement in Romans 15:13. The God of hope is not only the source but also the sustainer of hope. Your role in restoring hope is a partnership with the divine, and as you trust in Him, may you overflow with the transformative power of hope, bringing light to the lives you touch.

Journal:

1. Recall a specific patient or situation where you played a role in restoring hope. How did the experience impact you?

2. How does the concept of being filled with joy and peace as you trust in God relate to your ability to restore hope in your medical practice?

3. In what ways can you intentionally rely on the power of the Holy Spirit to overflow with hope in your interactions with patients and colleagues?

Day 6: The Calling to Serve

Verse of the Day:

Mark 10:45 (NIV) - "For even the Son of Man did not come to be served, but to serve, and to give his life as a ransom for many."

Reflection:

The essence of a medical profession is encapsulated in the profound words of Mark 10:45. It serves as a guiding light for every doctor, echoing the divine calling to serve selflessly. As you reflect on your vocation, recognize that you are partaking in a calling that aligns with the sacrificial nature of service exemplified by the Son of Man.

Consider the ways in which your daily work as a medical professional reflects the spirit of service. How does your commitment to the well-being of others echo the selflessness modeled by Jesus?

Reflect on the transformative power of service not only in the lives of those you care for but also in shaping your character and perspective as a healthcare provider. How has the act of serving impacted your personal and professional journey?

Encouragement:

In embracing the calling to serve, you emulate the very heart of Jesus. Your dedication to the well-being of others is a testament to the sacrificial love He demonstrated. May you find strength and fulfillment in knowing that your service is not in vain, echoing the eternal impact of Christ's selfless act.

Journal:

1. Share a specific instance where you felt a deep sense of fulfillment in serving others through your medical practice.

2. How does the calling to serve, as outlined in Mark 10:45, inspire and shape your approach to patient care?

3. Reflect on the challenges and rewards of embracing a life of service in your medical profession. How do you find spiritual and emotional fulfillment in your calling to serve?

Day 7: Balancing Science and Faith

Verse of the Day:

Proverbs 2:6 (NIV) - "For the Lord gives wisdom; from his mouth come knowledge and understanding."

Reflection:

In the intricate dance between science and faith, Proverbs 2:6 stands as a foundational truth. It affirms that true wisdom, knowledge, and understanding find their source in the divine. As a doctor navigating the realms of science and faith, reflect on the harmonious interplay of these two aspects in your life and profession.

Consider moments in your medical journey where the wisdom from God's mouth guided your decisions. How has the intersection of faith and medical knowledge shaped your practice?

Reflect on the depth of understanding that comes from seeking wisdom from the Lord. In what ways has this divine understanding influenced your approach to patient care, diagnosis, and treatment?

Encouragement:

As you balance the intricacies of science and faith, may you find assurance in the wisdom that comes from God. Your pursuit of knowledge, coupled with a foundation in faith, creates a powerful synergy that can impact not only the physical but also the spiritual well-being of those under your care.

Journal:

1. Share an experience where integrating your faith with medical knowledge brought about a unique perspective in patient care.

2. How do you navigate ethical dilemmas or challenging situations in your medical practice by drawing on the wisdom that comes from God?

3. Reflect on the ways in which your faith enhances your ability to connect with patients on a deeper level. How does this connection contribute to the overall healing process?

Day 8: Navigating Challenges

Verse of the Day:

Isaiah 41:10 (NIV) - "So do not fear, for I am with you; do not be dismayed, for I am your God. I will strengthen you and help you; I will uphold you with my righteous right hand."

Reflection:

The journey of a doctor is fraught with challenges and uncertainties. Isaiah 41:10 serves as a steadfast reminder of God's promise to be with you, to strengthen and uphold you in the midst of difficulties.

Reflect on how this assurance resonates with the challenges you face in your medical practice.

Consider moments in your career where you felt the weight of challenges. How did your faith provide a source of strength and comfort during these times?

Reflect on the ways God has upheld you with His righteous right hand.

Encouragement:

In the face of professional challenges, lean on the unwavering support of

God. His presence brings courage and strength, enabling you to navigate the complexities of medical practice. Find assurance in the promise that you are not alone, and God is actively involved in every aspect of your journey.

Journal:

1. Share a specific challenge you've encountered in your medical practice. How did you turn to God for strength and guidance during that time?

2. Reflect on the ways God has upheld you in your professional journey. Are there specific instances where you felt His presence and guidance in overcoming challenges?

3. Consider the uncertainties inherent in the field of medicine. How does the promise of God's presence and support influence your perspective on facing future challenges?

Day 9: The Healing Journey

Verse of the day:

Psalm 147:3 (NIV) - "He heals the brokenhearted and binds up their wounds."

Reflection:

In the intricate tapestry of the healing journey, Psalm 147:3 serves as a comforting reminder of God's role as the ultimate healer. As a doctor, reflect on the profound impact of this verse on your understanding of the healing process, both physically and emotionally.

Consider instances in your medical practice where you witnessed not only physical healing but also the binding of emotional wounds. How does recognizing God as the healer influence your approach to patient care?

Reflect on the correlation between healing and brokenness in the context of your profession. How can acknowledging God's role as the healer bring hope to those who are broken in body or spirit?

Encouragement:

As you embark on each healing journey, may the assurance that God heals the brokenhearted and binds up wounds inspire you. Your compassionate care becomes a reflection of the divine healing touch, bringing restoration to those entrusted to your medical expertise.

Journal:

1. Share a memorable experience where you witnessed the holistic healing of a patient, addressing both physical and emotional needs.

2. In what ways does acknowledging God as the ultimate healer impact your resilience and hope, especially during challenging cases or moments of loss?

3. Reflect on the role of empathy in your medical practice. How does expressing compassion contribute to the healing journey for both you and your patients?

Day 10: Resilience in Medicine

Verse of the Day:

Philippians 4:13 (NIV) - "I can do all this through him who gives me strength."

Reflection:

The journey of a medical professional is marked by challenges and uncertainties. In Philippians 4:13, find solace and empowerment, recognizing that your resilience in medicine is not solely dependent on personal strength but on the divine source of strength.

Reflect on instances in your medical career where you felt the need for resilience. How has relying on God's strength transformed your ability to navigate challenges in the field of medicine?

Consider the broader application of this verse in your life. In what ways can the strength provided by God extend beyond professional challenges to contribute to your overall well-being?

Encouragement:

In moments of exhaustion or when facing the complexities of medicine, remember that your resilience is deeply intertwined with God's strength. Embrace each challenge with the confidence that through Him, you can overcome and persevere.

Journal:

1. Share a specific challenge in your medical journey where you felt the need for resilience. How did relying on God's strength impact your response?

2. Reflect on the concept of resilience as not just professional but a holistic attribute. In what areas of your life do you desire God's strength to foster resilience?

3. Consider the impact of your resilience on those around you, including colleagues, patients, and loved ones. How can your reliance on God's strength inspire and encourage others?

Day 11: Compassionate Care

Verse of the Day:

Colossians 3:12 (NIV) - "Therefore, as God's chosen people, holy and dearly loved, clothe yourselves with compassion, kindness, humility, gentleness, and patience."

Reflection:

In the intricate tapestry of medical practice, compassion stands as a central thread, weaving together the diverse experiences of both healers and those seeking healing. Colossians 3:12 calls us, as God's chosen people, to adorn ourselves with qualities that include compassion. As a healthcare professional, your work is not merely a profession but a calling to embody God's love through compassionate care.

Consider the times when you've witnessed or experienced compassionate care in a medical setting. Reflect on how these moments, rooted in kindness and humility, left a lasting impact on both the giver and receiver of care. Compassion in healthcare extends beyond medical procedures; it touches the essence of human connection and empathy.

Encouragement:

Clothing ourselves with compassion is a divine directive, a reflection of God's own nature. In your medical journey, embrace the power of compassionate care as a transformative force. As you interact with patients, families, and colleagues, let compassion be a guiding principle, bringing healing not only to physical ailments but also to the deeper realms of the human spirit.

Journal:

1. Share a personal experience where you witnessed or received compassionate care in a medical setting. How did it impact the individuals involved?

2. Consider the challenges in maintaining compassion in the demanding field of medicine. How can you intentionally cultivate and express compassion in your daily interactions?

3. In what ways can you, as a healthcare professional, contribute to fostering a culture of compassion within your team or medical community?

Day 12: Guided Hands

Verse of the Day:

Isaiah 58:11 (NIV) - "The Lord will guide you always; he will satisfy your needs in a sun-scorched land and will strengthen your frame. You will be like a well-watered garden, like a spring whose waters never fail."

Reflection:

In the realm of medicine, where decisions can be weighty and paths unclear, the promise of divine guidance is a beacon of assurance. Isaiah 58:11 portrays a vivid image of God's continual guidance, satisfaction in barren circumstances, and the strengthening of one's essence. As a doctor, recognizing the source of your guidance is foundational to navigating the complexities of healthcare.

Take a moment to reflect on instances in your medical journey where you sensed divine guidance. Consider the times when decisions seemed challenging, and clarity emerged through a sense of assurance. Just as a well-watered garden flourishes, God's guidance ensures a fruitful and resilient professional journey.

Encouragement:

As a healthcare professional, your hands are instruments of healing guided by a higher wisdom. Embrace the truth that the Lord, who formed the intricacies of the human body, is also willing to guide your hands in the pursuit of health and wholeness. Trust in His leading, and find confidence in the promise that His guidance will sustain you even in the most challenging circumstances.

Journal:

1. Recall a specific moment in your medical practice where you felt a sense of divine guidance. How did this experience impact your decision-making and the outcomes for your patient?

2. In what ways do you currently seek guidance in your medical decisions? Reflect on how incorporating a reliance on God's guidance might enhance your professional journey.

3. Consider the challenges and uncertainties you currently face in your medical practice. How can you actively surrender these concerns to God, trusting in His guidance for the way forward?

45

Healing Hands, Guided Hearts: Daily Devotionals for Christian Doctors

Day 13: Embracing Vulnerability

Verse of the Day:

2 Corinthians 12:9 (NIV) - "But he said to me, 'My grace is sufficient for you, for my power is made perfect in weakness.' Therefore, I will boast all the more gladly about my weaknesses, so that Christ's power may rest on me."

Reflection:

Vulnerability is often seen as a weakness in the world, but 2 Corinthians 12:9 provides a profound perspective. It reminds us that in our weaknesses, Christ's power is perfected. As a doctor, acknowledging your vulnerabilities is not a sign of inadequacy but an invitation for divine strength to manifest in your healing ministry.

Reflect on moments in your medical career where you felt vulnerable or faced challenges. Consider how, in those moments, you experienced the sufficiency of God's grace. Embracing vulnerability allows Christ's transformative power to shine through, bringing hope and healing to both you and your patients.

Encouragement:

In a profession that demands resilience and strength, recognize that embracing vulnerability opens the door to a deeper experience of God's grace. Just as Christ's power rested on the Apostle Paul in his weaknesses, invite the same divine strength into your vulnerabilities. It is through acknowledging your limitations that you become a vessel for the extraordinary power of God.

Journal

1. Share a specific instance in your medical practice where you felt vulnerable or faced a challenge. How did you navigate through it, and what did you learn about God's grace in that situation?

2. Consider the cultural expectation for doctors to be strong and infallible. How can embracing vulnerability positively impact your well-being and the doctor-patient relationship?

3. Reflect on the connection between vulnerability and empathy in your interactions with patients. In what ways can acknowledging your own vulnerabilities enhance your ability to empathize with those under your care?

Day 14: The Gift of Discernment

Verse of the Day:

1 Corinthians 2:14 (NIV) - "The person without the Spirit does not accept the things that come from the Spirit of God but considers them foolishness, and cannot understand them because they are discerned only through the Spirit."

Reflection:

Discernment is a precious gift, especially in the intricate field of medicine. 1 Corinthians 2:14 emphasizes that spiritual discernment is a unique insight bestowed by the Holy Spirit. As a doctor, recognizing and cultivating this gift can lead to more profound insights into patient care, treatment plans, and overall well-being.

Reflect on instances in your medical journey where discernment played a crucial role. Consider times when you sensed a deeper understanding or insight that went beyond conventional knowledge. Acknowledge the role of the Holy Spirit in guiding your decisions and actions.

Encouragement:

Embrace the gift of discernment as you navigate the complexities of healthcare. It allows you to see beyond the surface, providing insights that may not be immediately apparent. Trust that the Holy Spirit, the ultimate source of discernment, is with you in every medical decision and interaction.

Journal:

1. Share a specific experience in your medical career where discernment played a significant role. How did it impact your decision-making and the well-being of your patient?

2. In what ways do you actively seek spiritual discernment in your medical practice? Are there specific practices or moments of reflection that enhance your sensitivity to the Holy Spirit's guidance?

3. Consider the challenges and ethical dilemmas in the field of medicine. How can the gift of discernment contribute to your ability to navigate these complexities with wisdom and compassion?

Day 15: Trusting the Divine Plan

Verse of the Day:

Proverbs 3:5-6 (NIV) - "Trust in the Lord with all your heart and lean not on your own understanding; in all your ways submit to him, and he will make your paths straight."

Reflection:

In the intricate tapestry of a doctor's journey, trust plays a pivotal role. Proverbs 3:5-6 offers a timeless reminder to place complete trust in the Lord, acknowledging that His understanding surpasses our own. As a doctor, entrusting your career, decisions, and even uncertainties to God can bring a profound sense of peace and assurance.

Reflect on moments in your medical career where trusting in God's plan made a difference. Consider instances where outcomes were beyond your control, and trusting in the divine plan brought clarity and purpose.

Encouragement:

Trusting in the divine plan allows you to navigate the complexities of medicine with confidence. As you submit your ways to the Lord, you invite His wisdom into every aspect of your medical practice. Embrace the assurance that God, in His infinite wisdom, is directing your path.

Journal:

1. Share a challenging situation in your medical career where trusting in God's plan brought peace or clarity. How did surrendering control impact your perspective?

2. In what ways do you currently seek God's guidance in your medical decisions and career choices? Are there areas where you can deepen your trust in His plan?

3. Consider the uncertainties and challenges in the field of medicine. How can trusting in the Lord's plan influence your approach to patient care, relationships with colleagues, and overall well-being?

Day 16: A Heart for Healing

Verse of the Day:

Ezekiel 36:26 (NIV) - "I will give you a new heart and put a new spirit in you; I will remove from you your heart of stone and give you a heart of flesh."

Reflection:

In the demanding realm of medicine, maintaining a compassionate and empathetic heart is vital. Ezekiel 36:26 beautifully illustrates God's transformative power, emphasizing the renewal of our hearts. As a doctor, nurturing a heart of flesh in the face of challenges ensures not only your well-being but also the well-being of those under your care.

Reflect on the condition of your heart in your medical practice. Consider moments when compassion prevailed, and contemplate instances where the challenges may have hardened your heart.

Encouragement:

God's promise to give a new heart is an invitation to seek His grace for emotional and spiritual resilience. Embrace the promise of a heart of flesh, allowing God's love to flow through you in your role as a healer.

Journal:

1. Recall a specific patient interaction where you felt your heart was deeply moved. How did that experience impact your approach to medical care?

2. In challenging and demanding situations, do you find your heart becoming hardened or more compassionate? How can the promise of a new heart in Ezekiel 36:26 influence your response to difficulties?

3. Consider practical ways to cultivate a heart of flesh in your medical practice. How can you intentionally foster empathy, compassion, and a healing presence in your interactions with patients and colleagues?

57

Day 17: Gratitude in Service

Verse of the Day:

1 Thessalonians 5:18 (NIV) - "Give thanks in all circumstances; for this is God's will for you in Christ Jesus."

Reflection:

In the journey of a medical professional, cultivating gratitude is a transformative practice. 1 Thessalonians 5:18 encourages an attitude of thanksgiving in all circumstances. As a doctor, embracing gratitude in your service not only fosters personal well-being but also amplifies the impact of your healing ministry.

Reflect on moments in your medical career where gratitude played a role. Consider the challenges and victories, recognizing the significance of maintaining a thankful heart.

Encouragement:

Gratitude is a powerful force that can shift perspectives and bring joy even in the midst of trials. As you serve others, let thankfulness be a guiding light, illuminating the blessings within the challenges and the privilege of making a positive impact on lives.

Journal:

1. Recall a challenging situation in your medical practice where gratitude helped you navigate through difficulties. How did a thankful mindset influence the outcome?

2. In what ways can you incorporate intentional gratitude into your daily routine as a medical professional? How might this practice impact your overall well-being and the atmosphere of your workplace?

3. Consider the broader scope of your medical service. How does gratitude align with your calling to serve others? How can cultivating gratitude enhance your effectiveness as a healer?

Day 18: Wisdom for Diagnosis

Verse of the Day:

James 1:5 (NIV) - "If any of you lacks wisdom, you should ask God, who gives generously to all without finding fault, and it will be given to you."

Reflection:

In the intricate world of medicine, the quest for wisdom is paramount. James 1:5 reminds us that divine wisdom is accessible to those who seek it. For doctors, the ability to diagnose accurately requires not only knowledge but a wisdom that transcends human understanding.

Reflect on instances where seeking divine wisdom influenced your medical decisions. Consider the complexity of diagnoses and the role of God's wisdom in guiding your discernment.

Encouragement:

As you navigate the challenges of diagnosis, lean on God's promise to generously provide wisdom. Trust that His insight goes beyond textbooks and charts, offering a divine perspective that can lead to more profound understanding and effective treatment.

Journal:

1. Recall a specific case where you sought wisdom in making a diagnosis. How did relying on God's guidance impact your decision-making process?

2. In what ways do you currently integrate prayer or seeking divine wisdom into your medical practice? How might a more intentional incorporation of this spiritual discipline enhance your ability to diagnose and treat patients?

3. Wisdom often comes through a combination of experience and divine insight. How do you balance the knowledge gained through medical education with seeking God's wisdom in your daily practice?

Day 19: Endurance in Healing

Verse of the Day:

Romans 15:5 (NIV) - "May the God who gives endurance and encouragement give you the same attitude of mind toward each other that Christ Jesus had."

Reflection:

In the journey of healing, endurance is often a virtue doctors must embody. Romans 15:5 speaks of God as the source of endurance and encouragement. Reflect on the challenges you face in the healing process and how God's endurance sustains you.

Consider instances where your endurance was tested in the pursuit of healing for your patients. How has your mindset toward endurance been influenced by the example of Christ Jesus?

Encouragement:

As you encounter the ebb and flow of healing, draw strength from the well of divine endurance. Just as Christ exemplified steadfastness, trust that God's endurance will empower you to persevere in your healing ministry.

Journal:

1. Recall a challenging case where endurance played a significant role in the healing process. How did your faith and reliance on God's endurance impact your approach?

2. In what ways do you currently seek endurance in your medical practice? How might a deeper connection with God's enduring strength influence your resilience as a healer?

3. Reflect on Christ's attitude of mind towards others. How can you emulate this attitude in your interactions with patients, colleagues, and those involved in the healing journey?

Day 20: Rest for the Weary

Verse of the Day:

Matthew 11:28 (NIV) - "Come to me, all you who are weary and burdened, and I will give you rest."

Reflection:

In the demanding field of medicine, weariness can become a companion. Matthew 11:28 extends a comforting invitation from Jesus to find rest. Reflect on moments of weariness in your medical journey and how you've sought rest in Christ.

Consider the burdens you carry, both professionally and personally. How does the promise of rest in Matthew 11:28 resonate with the challenges you face in your role as a healer?

Encouragement:

Amidst the demands of your profession, find solace in Christ's offer of rest. Recognize that seeking rest is not a sign of weakness but a wise and rejuvenating choice. Embrace the rest Jesus provides for the weary soul.

Journal:

1. Identify specific instances in your medical career where weariness became pronounced. How did you cope with these moments, and were there times when you sought rest in Christ?

2. Explore the concept of rest in both a physical and spiritual context. How can finding rest in Christ contribute to your overall well-being as a healthcare professional?

3. In what practical ways can you incorporate moments of rest and rejuvenation into your daily or weekly routine? How might prioritizing rest positively impact your effectiveness as a healer?

69

Day 21: The Light of Compassion

Verse of the Day:

Matthew 5:16 (NIV) - "In the same way, let your light shine before others, that they may see your good deeds and glorify your Father in heaven."

Reflection:

As you conclude this devotional series for doctors, ponder the significance of being a light in the world of medicine. Reflect on how Matthew 5:16 guides you to shine a compassionate light through your healing work.

Consider instances where your deeds as a healthcare professional have impacted others. How can your daily actions in the medical field become a beacon of God's love and compassion?

Encouragement:

Embrace the calling to be a light in your profession. Your compassion and care have the power to illuminate the lives of those you serve. May your medical practice be a testimony that glorifies the Father in heaven.

Journal:

1. Recall specific moments in your medical career where you've witnessed the positive impact of your actions on others. How do these instances align with the concept of being a light in Matthew 5:16?

2. In what ways can you intentionally let your light shine in your daily interactions with patients, colleagues, and others in the medical community? How might this contribute to a culture of compassion in your workplace?

3. As you move forward in your medical journey, how will you continue to be a source of light and compassion? What steps can you take to ensure that your professional practice glorifies your Father in heaven?

Conclusion

In this journey of devotionals tailored for doctors, we have delved into the intricate tapestry of a medical professional's life—a life of healing, compassion, and unwavering commitment. Each day has been an exploration of the spiritual dimensions intertwined with the noble calling to serve others through the practice of medicine.

As you conclude this collection, take a moment to appreciate the sacred dance between the art and science of healing. Your hands, guided by skill and knowledge, become instruments of God's grace in the lives of those entrusted to your care. The divine verses have illuminated the path, offering peace, wisdom, and encouragement to fortify your steps.

Reflect on the profound responsibility carried by healing hands. From embracing the divine gift of healing to navigating challenges, seeking wisdom, and embodying resilience, you've embarked on a spiritual odyssey that resonates with the heartbeat of your vocation. The divine diagnoses you make, the hope you restore, and the compassionate care you provide are not mere actions but reflections of a calling deeply rooted in love.

The pages of this devotional series echo the heartbeat of compassion, guiding you to find strength, wisdom, and endurance in the embrace of God's word. As you stand at the intersection of science and faith, may the light of compassion continue to shine brightly through your endeavors, impacting lives and glorifying the Father in heaven.

In the continuous ebb and flow of the medical journey, may you find gratitude in service, endurance in healing, and rest for the weary. May your heart, now tenderized by the divine touch, carry the wisdom of Proverbs, the love of Corinthians, and the resilience of Philippians into the realms of medicine.

And so, as you step forward into the healing spaces of each new day, may the divine wisdom you've gleaned from these devotionals serve as a lamp unto your feet and a light unto your path. For in nurturing the healer's heart, you not only fulfill a noble profession but live out a sacred calling that transcends the boundaries of science and touches the very soul of humanity.

With warmest wishes and gratitude,

Delightful Devotionals